SUSAN BROUGHER

WANT TO
Feel Better—
KEEP LAVENDER HANDY

Essential Oils, Energy, Safety, Support

outskirts press

"This book is a great resource guide, whether you're a beginner wanting to learn and dabble in essential oils or much more seasoned in the field. I can tell that a lot of research has gone into this book. It offers so many thought- provoking passages throughout. Susan encourages people to live better through plants. She inspires, educates, promotes wellness, and encourages love. I feel it throughout the entire book. Aww, I can smell the lavender!" *Kathy Pyle, Aroma Therapies Spa, Owner, Esthetician, Therapist, Herbalist, Somerset, PA*

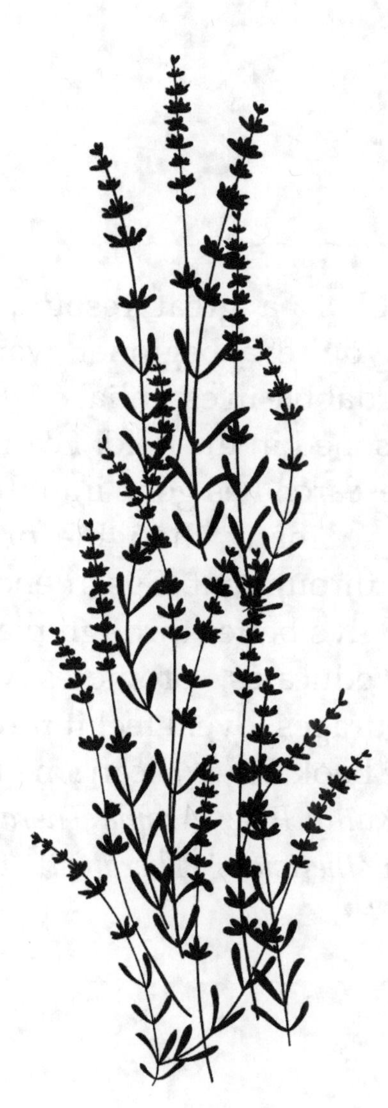

Books by Susan Brougher

The Strongest Bond, a memoir about coming of age without a mother for guidance.

The Magic of Christmas-The Magic of Love, illustrated poems for children and the young at heart.

The Magical Kingdom of Ing, an enchanting tale of fairies and dragons.

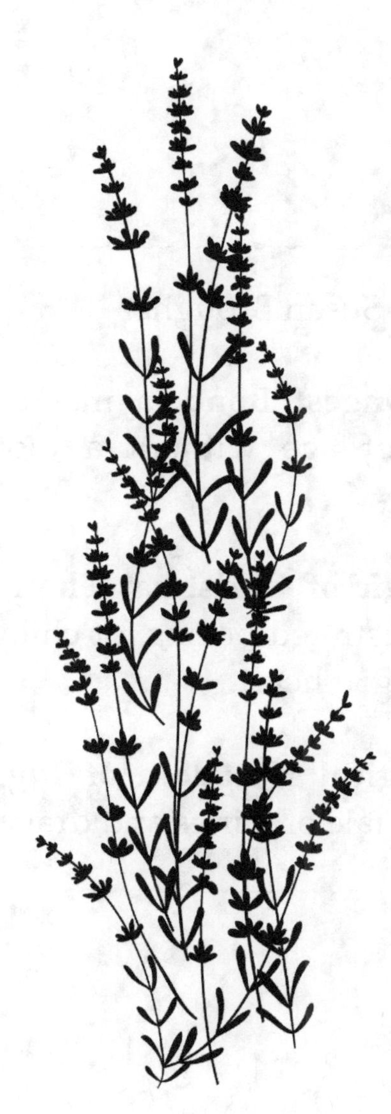

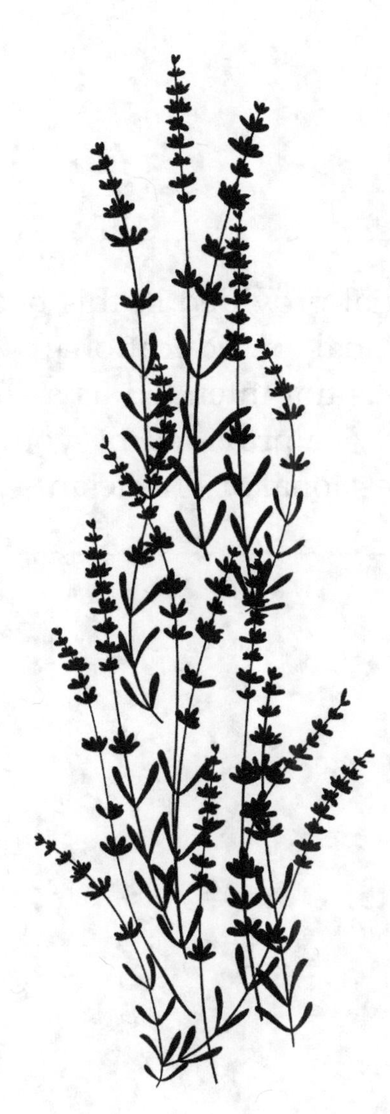

Live in each season as it passes; breathe the air, drink the drink, taste the fruit, and resign yourself to the influence of the earth.

~ Henry David Thoreau

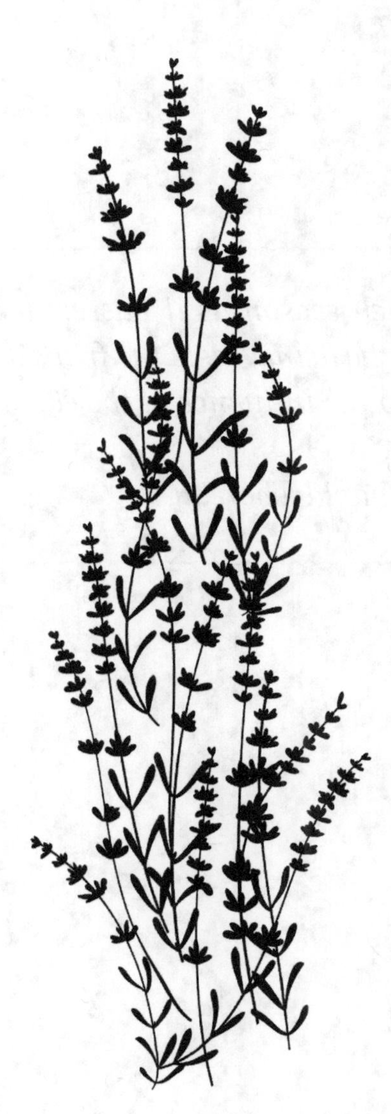

TABLE OF CONTENTS

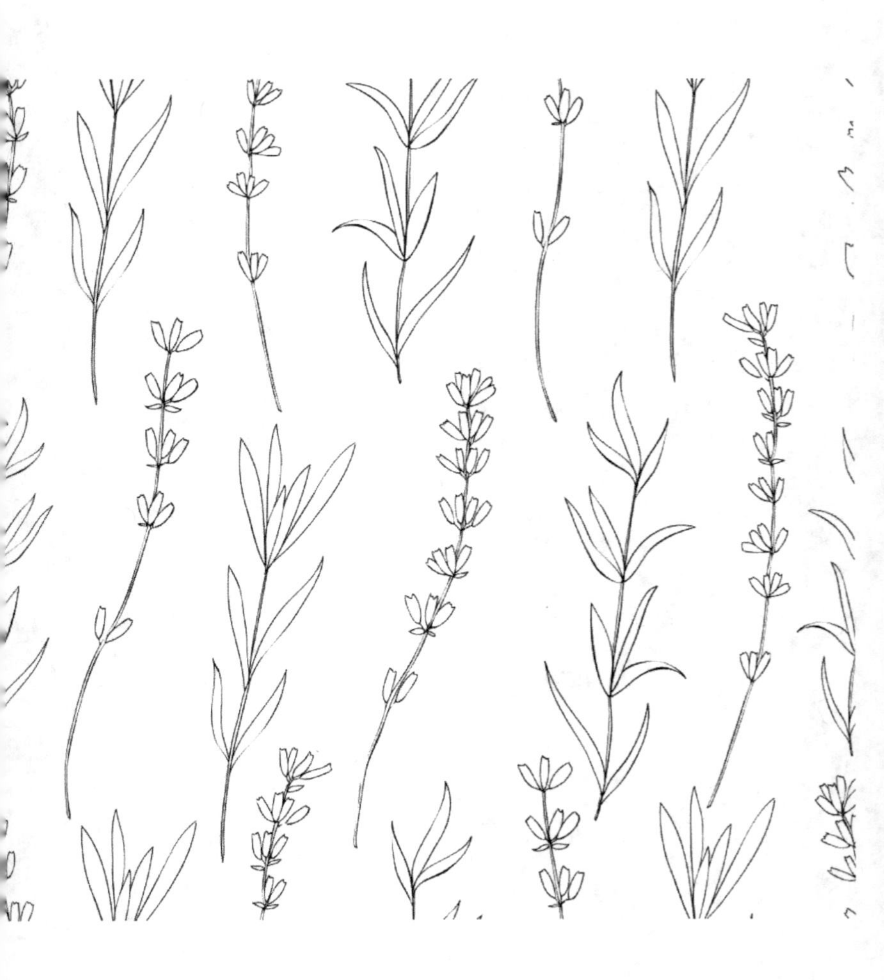

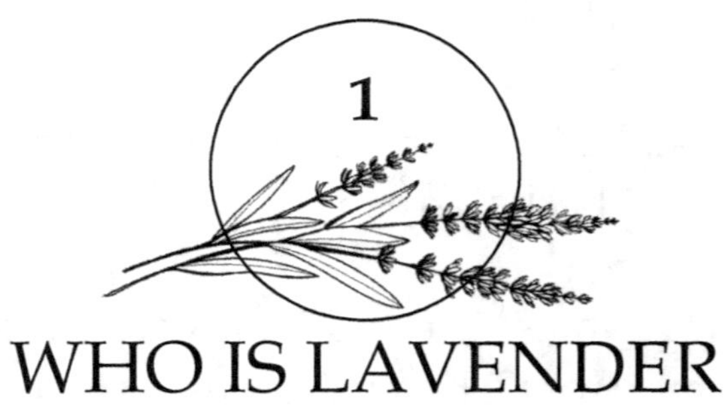

WHO IS LAVENDER

"It always seems to me as if the lavender was a little woman in a green dress, with a lavender bonnet and a white kerchief. She's one of those strong, sweet, wholesome people, who always rest you, and her sweetness lingers long after she goes away."

Myrtle Reed

To meet lavender is to breathe her magical, sweet, floral and herbal aroma. Lavender helps your skin, muscles, joints, and nerves. She enters your everyday life to improve sleep, reduce stress, and lift depression. When lavender's essential oil is distilled from the freshly cut flowering tops, she is a floral. When the leafy stalks are distilled with the flowers, she is an herbal green.

What is an essential oil, and where does it come from? Essential oils come from plants, although not all plants yield essential oils. They are produced in tiny sacs or canals within the plant's cells in different parts of the plant. Essential oil odors attract pollinators and can repel predators wanting to nibble on them.

Magic can be described as the movement of subtle, natural energies to bring about a change. Plants radiate nature's energy by releasing their scents for us to enjoy. The moment we bend to pick a flower, the magic begins.

Down through history the Greek, Chinese, and many other cultures believed in the energy of the elements. The five traditional elements are wood, fire, earth, metal (air), and water. The air element relates to the heavenly bodies and spirit. Lavender is associated with the element of air, which reminds us of our true divine self and takes us beyond our conflicts and into harmony.

If you have a lavender personality, you might feel like there are days when you're filled with floral energy, loving how you look and how people are looking at you. On those herbal days, you will want to love and be loved.

Other essential oils take advantage of lavender's ability to increase their power. This happens when lavender is added to the group in therapeutic blends. It is the ever-present helper who never tries to overpower beautiful florals like rose or strong herbals like peppermint. Lavender is like a middle child who manages to get along with everyone.

Among its many variations or species, the lavender angustifolia, or true lavender, stands out as a high-quality healer.

Lavender's name came from the Latin word *lavare,* meaning to wash. Down through history it was widely used as a toilet water. This makes it sound ordinary, but it is not. Lavender comes from the Labiatae or Lamiaceae family of mint flowering plants. The fancy family name suits lavender since it is a worldwide cosmopolitan traveler, spreading aromas into many areas.

Most people are familiar with what lavender looks like because it is so popular. Lavender cares about her appearance and is easy on the eyes with strong yet beautiful features. This aromatic evergreen stands about 3 feet tall with lance-shaped leaves and purple flowers that bees buzz about.

Lavender grew up by the sea in a Mediterranean climate with mild rainy winters and hot dry summers. No wonder lavender is so calm and relaxing. Many essential oils of lavender are produced in Bulgaria and France.

Do you know caring and compassionate people? Are they nurses or teachers? Then you might know a lavender person. Mailhebiau, a French author, compared lavender to Mother Teresa: "Tireless, always even-tempered, with unfailing gentleness and devotion. Lavender cares for and calms, listens to, and remedies a thousand ills. She takes care of children, adults and elderly, animals, plants, the earth and sky. She looks after everyone with equal love and if there is anyone in the world whom she neglects, it is herself."

The *Doctrine of the Signatures* is like an autograph or personality. Healing properties of plants are influenced by their inherited physical features and their environment. The makeup of a plant's shape, texture, and color tells us about its actions.

For example, in aromatherapy it is valuable to consider the shape of the whole plant that produces the essential oil. A strong tree that reaches upward is different from a gentle rose hanging on a vine. A flower's soft delicate nature is revealed in a floral essential oil. The violet-colored flowers of true lavender reflect a calm, spiritual nature.

The parts of a plant disclose the nature of its personality. Roots ground and stabilize. Wood steadies and strengthens. Flowers attract and reproduce. Leaves breathe like lungs. Fruits protect and nurture. Resins soothe and rest. And seeds invigorate and digest.

Lavender's story down through history:

Lavender was used for mummification and fragrance. Royal families and high priests used it for cosmetic and medicinal purposes.

Cleopatra, Queen of the Nile, anointed her body with lavender oil to seduce Julius Caesar and Mark Anthony.

The Greek philosopher Diogenes felt lavender applied to the head flies into the air for the birds. Instead it should be rubbed on the lower limbs for the whole body to enjoy.

Roman soldiers carried lavender to dress war wounds.

Pliny the Elder, a Greek writer, listed lavender as helping menstrual problems, upset stomachs, kidney disorders, and insect bites.

Hildegard of Bingen, an author of theology, botany, and medicines, wrote that lavender oil was effective in treating head lice and fleas.

During the Renaissance in 16th century France, glove makers perfumed their wares with lavender. They often escaped being infected with the cholera bacteria, which caused fatal intestinal disease.

In Medieval Europe, lavender was used to scent drawers. Women dried laundry on lavender bushes. And even today you can find lavender-scented paper drawer liners.

In the Middle Ages, Queen Elizabeth used it in her tea for frequent migraines and as a perfume.

By the 16th century, lavender was established as the "herb of cleanliness and calm."

In the 18th century, Empress Josephine, the wife of Napoleon Bonaparte, used lavender as a powerful aphrodisiac to arouse sexual desire. Did she give Napoleon a shot of lavender in his hot chocolate when going to bed, maybe?

Queen Victoria was a lavender enthusiast. Lavender appeared in the London Pharmacopeia, but by the 20th century it had lost appeal due to its association with old ladies.

Rene Gattefosse, a founder of modern-day aromatherapy, verified the healing and antiseptic powers of lavender after badly burning his hand while working in his lab. He quickly applied lavender oil, causing the pain to stop and the burn to heal without becoming infected or scarred.

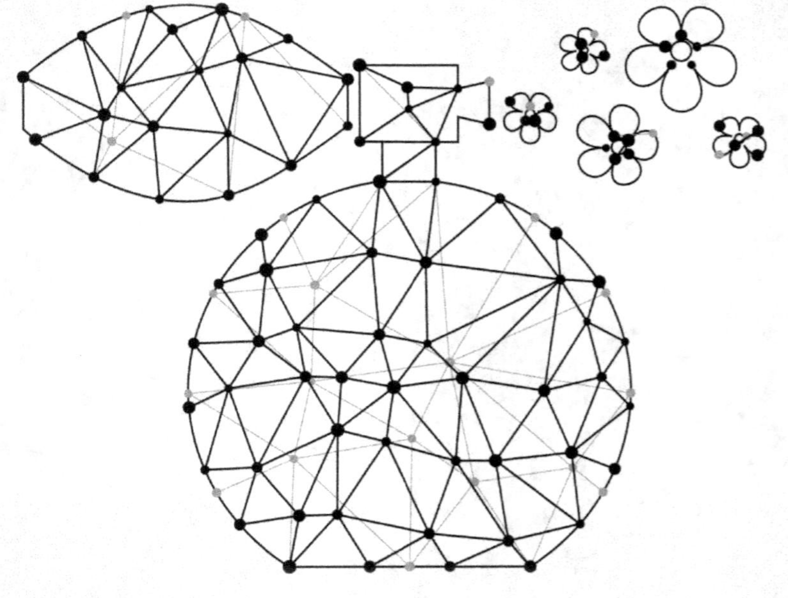

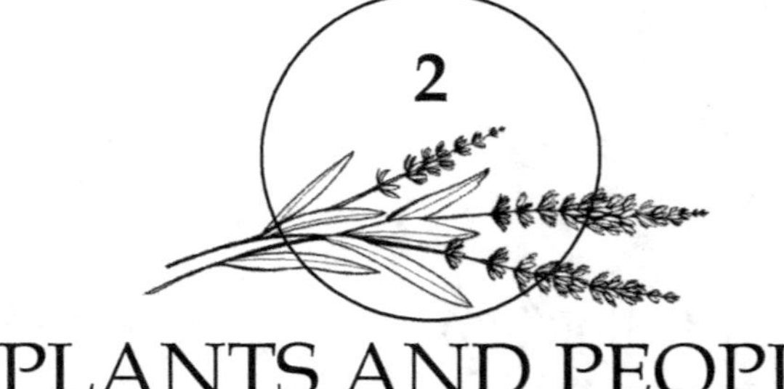

PLANTS AND PEOPLE

"When nothing else subsists from the past, after the people are dead, after the things are broken and scattered … the smell and taste of things remain poised a long time, like souls … bearing resiliently, on tiny and almost impalpable drops of their essence, the immense edifice of memory."

Marcel Proust

Want to learn more about this popular purple plant? Unravel your own links to lavender. It is the essential oil of comfort that brings a scent of balance to all it touches. Fall in love with lavender or decide you don't like her. Either way, she will grace you with her natural splendor and give her life-essence for your healing.

The word "link" points to a relationship between two things, especially when one thing touches the other. A link or connection could easily exist between people and plants. The origin of the word link dates back to the 16th century, perhaps from medieval Latin li(n)chinus or "wick" and from the Greek lukhnos, "light," meaning a torch for lighting the way in dark streets. If this is so, finding your link to lavender should be enlightening. Essential oils connect to nature's energy and radiate a natural perfume for life, a link between us and the universe.

Lavender has many therapeutic actions. It is analgesic (pain relieving), antidepressant, antispasmodic (cramp relieving), antiseptic (destroying disease causing bacteria), antiviral, decongestant, hypotensive (blood pressure lowering), and sedative, to mention a few of its qualities.

Lavender has been used successfully in many clinical trials in hospitals as a massage oil, vaporized for helping anxiety, and it has been shown to decrease the need for drugs to help patients sleep.

Aromatherapy or essential oil therapy is the art and science of using aromatic plants for holistic healing to balance soul, mind, and body. Traditional medicine views the word "body" as physical. A holistic approach interprets the word "body" as spiritual, emotional, mental, and physical. On a scale of 1 to 10, with 1 being the least like you and 10 the most like you, note your score then add for a total. By doing this simple assessment you can discover your own link to lavender. Give it a try.

SOUL (SPIRITUAL & EMOTIONAL)	SCORE
Kind	
Intuitive	

Balanced	
Honest	
Nourishing	
Total	
A score from 35 to 50 could indicate a lavender personality. Even so, you may still enjoy using it to boost your natural tendencies. A lower score may indicate a need or desire to enhance these qualities by using lavender. Each person's reaction to the smell of lavender will be different. It's possible to have several lavender soul traits but not like the smell of lavender.	
MIND (MENTAL)	
Anxious	
Irritable	
Depressed	
Sleepless	
Stressed	
Total	

A score from 30 to 50 could indicate a need for lavender to ease your mind and help you relax. A lower score may indicate that your mind is not often bothered by these symptoms, but if you have occasional problems sleeping or feel stressed, lavender can help.	
BODY (PHYSICAL)	
Bite/Bruise/Rash/Itch	
Palpitations	
Aches & Pains	
High Blood Pressure	
Headaches	
Total	
A score from 25 to 50 could indicate a need for lavender to bring you comfort. A lower score may mean these symptoms occur once in a while. But if you experience occasional heart palpitations or headaches, lavender could be used to help calm your heart and relieve your headache.	

A plant's essential oil is akin to the blood that runs through our veins. It is a life force. As I studied and applied essential oils, I began to see how their unique qualities matched my client's character and needs. People either loved or hated a particular aroma. Smells do matter.

Speculation has it that "plants might be people too," sort of like "pets are people too." They may know and feel more than we've imagined. See what you think after reading this classic Backster experiment performed years ago involving plant murder. Cleve Backster began his career as an Interrogation Specialist with the Central Intelligence Agency (CIA). He founded the CIA's polygraph unit shortly after World War II.

Mr. Backster placed two plants next to each other in a room with six of his students. Each student drew a piece of paper from a hat. One piece of paper had instructions to murder. Backster and the students with the five blank pieces of paper left the room. The student with instructions to murder stayed and ripped one of the plants to shreds.

The remaining unharmed plant was then attached to a polygraph machine. The students returned to the room one by one. There was no response on the machine to the five innocent students. But when the murderer entered, the pen flew across the paper. The unharmed plant or the silent witness recognized the guilty student.

Plants know things. Who says talking to plants is foolish? Give them kind words of love, and they in turn grow green leaves and bright flowers to warm your heart. You wouldn't want them telling anyone how close they came to dying from dehydration because you forgot to water them.

According to a June 2020 article in *The EPOCH Times* by Tatiana Denning, DO, a family medicine physician, "IKEA conducted an informally scientific study in a school in United Arab Emirates to show the effects of unkind words on plants, with the goal of encouraging kids not to bully one another by saying unkind things. Two plants were kept in identical conditions, with plant 'A' being subjected to bullying words, and the other complimented. After 30 days, the bullied plant was wilted and noticeably droopy while the complimented plant was thriving." Plants show us how they feel when mistreated, and they help us to teach our children the importance of kind, positive words.

We have learned from recent studies that plants can talk to each other, so why not to us? When you're quiet and listen closely, you may hear them. Research has shown that plants communicate with each other to warn of danger. Flowers don't cry when you cut them, but that does not mean they aren't screaming in a chemical language at a decibel range we can't hear. They release compounds into the air to help their neighbors by chemically warning of disease so other plants can mount a defense. Plants are like people; they look out for each other.

my dreams

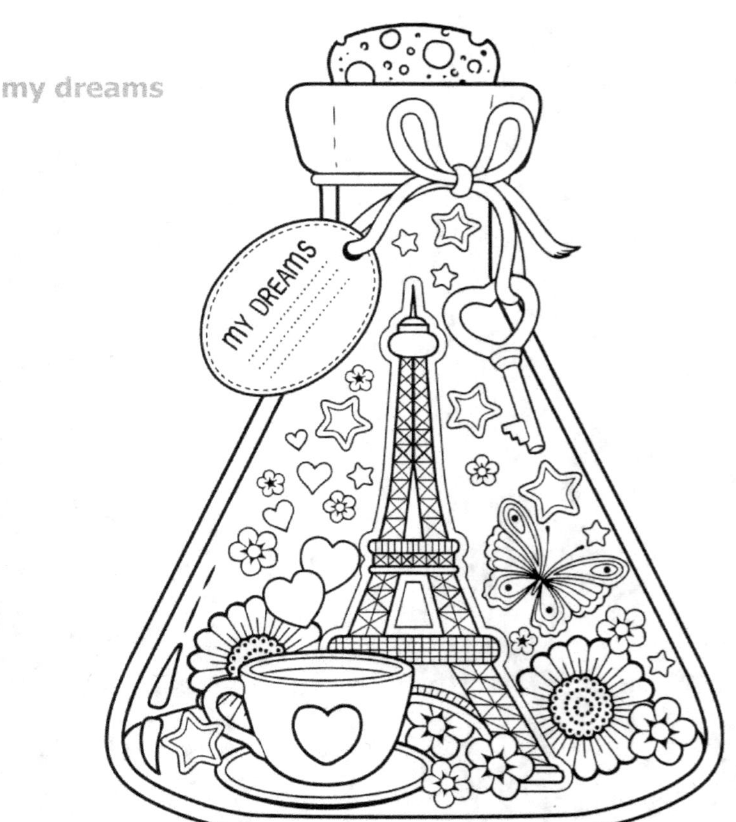
MY DREAMS

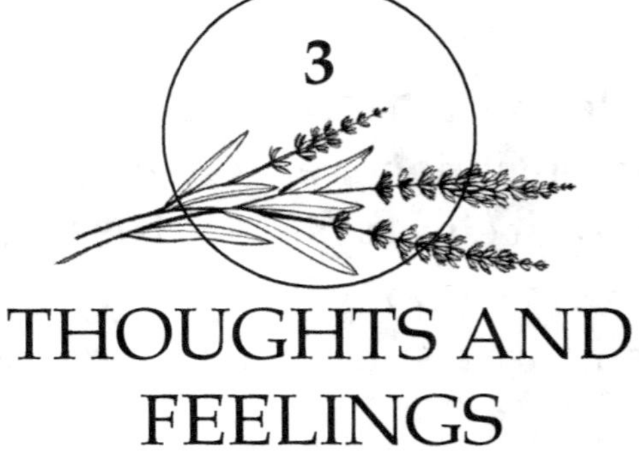

THOUGHTS AND FEELINGS

"The cure of the part should not be attempted without treatment of the whole, and also no attempt should be made to cure the body without the soul, and therefore if the head and body are to be well you must begin by curing the mind: that is the first thing... for this is the error of our day in the treatment of the human body, that physicians separate the soul from the body."

Plato, Chronicles

Lavender is a medicine for the soul, as are most plants and the essential oils they produce. They offer us the ability to integrate spirit into our being. An energy healing practitioner expressed an unusual way of seeing a person. He said, "We think we are a body walking a spirit, but we really are a spirit walking a body."

We often think of ourselves as more body then spirit or soul. It may be because our solid body is easy to observe, study, and define. Many years in nursing, caring for people with ailing bodies, taught me that patients had an ever-present spirit. In fact, nursing may be more about nurturing souls then it is about restoring bodies.

My childhood was rich with nature's soul-stirring scents. The best way to describe this is to share a passage from my first book, *The Strongest Bond*, a memoir about coming of age without a mother to guide me. She died of cancer when I was fourteen. "The old dead branches beneath the pine formed a roof covering. An earthen floor of cool dirt, roots, leaves, and pine needles rested under my feet. Their strong earthy aromas encircled every part of my being and tucked me away from the rest of the world." Nature can soothe hurting, give comfort, and build your strength with its green grassy fields, a creek, and a tall old pine tree to sit beneath.

Light travels in the form of a wave. We sense these waves as color. Red is the slowest vibration and has the longest wavelength. The life-force energy of red is reflected in the color of our blood and our physical body. Violet is the fastest vibration and has the shortest wavelength. Violet and blue can be said to connect us to the heavens and to our higher mind or soul.

Visible light is the range of wavelengths that the eye responds to or sees. Our blood and body fluids move in sympathy with certain wavelengths of color. Each of these colored rays has its own health-giving action.

The color frequency of violet or lavender corresponds to the pineal gland, the head, spine, central nervous system, and our psyche. The pineal gland is a small pinecone-shaped endocrine organ. It sits alone in the middle of the brain and at the same level as the eyes. Descartes, a famous philosopher, described it as the "principal seat of the soul." You may have heard it referred to as the "third eye," a mystical point right in the middle of your eyebrows.

How we think and feel every day is dependent on our pineal gland. It produces the hormone melatonin, which influences the quality and length of our sleep. This tiny organ regulates the daily seasonal sleep-wake patterns that determine our hormone and stress levels.

How does one define those puzzling things we call emotions? We touch, hear, taste, see, and smell. And what about our not easily defined sixth sense that gives us the ability to perceive the subtle or elusive unseen?

Our senses allow us to figure out what is going on by feeding information to the nervous system. It is our communication network that picks up changes, interprets them, and responds with action. When we have an emotional or mental aliment, it is not uncommon to become sick in our physical body.

It is here, in dealing with our mind and emotions that essential oils offer multifaceted healing. Did you know that odors are rarely if ever forgotten by us and can strongly impact our emotions? Have you been transported in an instant by a smell that brought back memories of a loved one? Have you inhaled an aroma that reminded you of something, but you didn't know what? Did it make you feel sad or happy? According to Heinrich Heine, "Perfumes are the feelings of flowers."

We draw smells up into the yellowish patch in the roof of our nose when we inhale. It contains fifty million receptor cells with microscopic hairs that connect directly to our brain on a long nerve fiber. This tells us how important smell is, yet it is something we often take for granted. Recorded studies have shown that an electroencephalogram (an electronic reading of brain waves) demonstrated that smelling lavender stimulated alpha or dominant waves in the brain and caused relaxation.

This olfactory area of our brain is part of the limbic system or the "smell brain." We know the limbic system is connected to our instinctive drives, for example emotion, intuition, memory, creativity, sleep, hunger, thirst, and our sex drive. It's pretty significant and mystifying.

A healthy sense of smell means we are able to detect over ten thousand different odors. Why not make lavender one of them? It can help to restore the rest and balance needed for sound sleep. It is perfect for a mind that is constantly filling with new ideas, ever searching, learning, and looking for things to do. According to traditional Chinese medicine, anxiety is linked to the heart, or the home of the mind.

Today, lavender enjoys a list of uses that exert a positive influence on our emotions. Lavender will come to you when you feel rotten. It soothes aching joints, quiets coughs, and chases the germs away. We take our bodies everywhere we go, inside sitting at the computer or outside walking the dog. Our body is ours to live in. We need to keep it healthy to enjoy our life.

Lavender is so confident and comfortable with itself that it is powerful alone or when mixed with other essential oils where it amplifies the blend. It is an exceptional natural first aid remedy. Carry a 10 milliliter (ml) roll-on of undiluted lavender with you. It's helpful to dab on cuts, bumps, bruises, and bug bites. Indoors, it's handy in the kitchen for nicks and burns. Roll it on fingertips as an antiseptic when out and about with no access to handwashing facilities.

Keep a spray bottle of lavender mixed in distilled water in the refrigerator for a refreshing spray toner. Use it for your dog if they are nervous when going to the veterinarian. Fluff it in their hair to keep bugs away, and to make it shine. Cool pets off on hot days. When that final day comes to say goodbye to your pet, use it to comfort your pet and yourself.

On a well-labeled bottle of lavender essential oil you will find: company name and contact data such as an email or mailing address, the essential oils common name, country of origin, for example Lavender (Bulgaria), and genus and species (Lavandula angustifolia). Essential oil should be the only ingredient listed. It should also have the amount, for example 100 ml (3.3 fl oz), the lot number, and that it is not for internal use.

When you incorporate essential oils into your lifestyle, your health will improve. It is challenging to control life's stressors. But you can control how you respond to them by using essential oils for holistic support. It makes a difference. Listen to the soulful mourning dove and let summer breezes stir your hair and the drifting fragrance of lavender fill your head with long-forgotten thoughts.

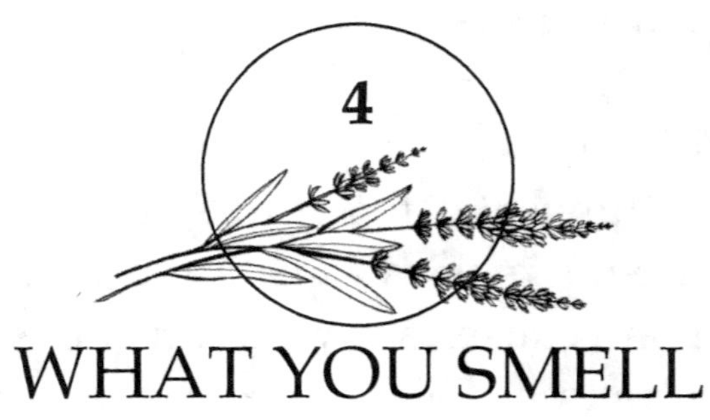

WHAT YOU SMELL

"It is more important to know what sort of person has a disease than to know what sort of disease a person has. Cure sometimes, treat often, comfort always. Natural forces within us are the true healers of disease."

Hippocrates

It is said that we could close our eyes to beauty and to horrors, and our ears to lovely melodies or to ugly words. But we cannot escape scent. Together with breath it entered us humans, for to breathe is to live.

It's easy to take our sense of smell for granted and hard to imagine what it would be like not to smell even the stinky things. Losing your sense of smell is a serious malady called anosmia. The two main causes are viral infections and head trauma. Did you know the complete loss of smell can result in depression? We continually smell but may not notice these aromas as they weave their way into our lives.

Have you ever wondered why you are drawn to one aroma over another? Your sense of smell is directly connected to your emotions. Think about it. Why do you wear a certain perfume? Is it to feel good because you smell good? Does the essential oil or perfume aroma you choose match your physical and emotional character? Or is the aroma you select needed to balance what is absent in your health and temperament?

There is a profound connection between the sense of smell and your brain. Fragrance research has discovered that odors influence your mood, fight stress, and decrease blood pressure.

In the Middle Ages, medical theory suggested the nose gave direct access to the brain. They believed inhalation moved the spirit or life force to correct disorders. Physicians called for sickrooms to have herbs at the window, an aromatic fire burning in the fireplace, and rosewater and vinegar sprinkled on the floor. Could you envision an order for that now in our hospitals? Maybe not such a bad idea.

Doctors often wore a nose-bag, a comical-looking long beak over their nose to breathe. The beak was filled with cinnamon, cloves, and aromatic herbs and was designed to protect them from putrid air, which was seen as the cause of infection. You can find fascinating images of the doctor's clothing on Google by typing "plague mask."

Essential oils provide powerful germ-killing properties. According to a 2016 article in *Evidence-based Complementary and Alternative Medicine*, "Essential oils have great potential in the field of biomedicine as they effectively destroy several bacterial, fungal, and viral pathogens." More study is needed in this area due to the increase in antibiotic-resistant pathogens.

Did you know that in France in the late 1800s it was realized that some essential oils were extremely antimicrobial or able to resist or destroy germs? The incidence of tuberculosis (TB) was low in the flower-growing districts in France, especially in the south. At that time, TB was a common illness. It was noted that most workers who processed the flowers and herbs were free of respiratory diseases.

So why does it matter if you have a link to lavender or if plants really are like people? Plants, through history, have been healers, and their power remains important to our emotional and physical health today. Can you hear lavender whispering, "Sit back, relax, and take a deep breath."

Essential oils carry electrical charges helpful to healing. They are energetic and produce electricity at megahertz (MHz) frequencies, the radio frequency range, or millions of cycles per second. All cells communicate with one another through vibrational impulses that can flow between organisms. When we meet people, there is an exchange of energy. If a person's vibrations are in sympathy with your own, you tend to like them, and when a person's vibrations are not in sync with yours, they tend to "get on your nerves." Sound familiar?

Energy can be expressed as an electromagnetic vibrational frequency. Electromagnetic energy is a form of energy reflected or emitted from objects via electrical or magnetic waves traveling through space. Everything vibrates. Every atom in the universe has a specific vibratory motion.

Essential oils are a mixture of divine, pulsing molecules. Their chemistry is so diverse and complex that for example, rose essential oil has over 300 chemical compounds, of which many are yet to be identified. Essential oil components all contain carbon, hydrogen, and at times, oxygen.

Most of the human body is made up of water. Our cells are 65-90% water by weight. Carbon is 18%, hydrogen is 10%, and oxygen is 65%. These three elements, plus nitrogen, make up most living things.

Carbon is the basic building block required to form proteins, carbohydrates, and fats, and it plays a crucial role in regulating physiology, or body makeup. Hydrogen in the body is mostly bound with oxygen to form water. Hydrogen acts as a proton or positive ion in chemical reactions. An ion is a group of atoms or particles with an electrical charge. Oxygen plays a critical role in the body. It is used to oxidize our food, thus releasing energy. Oxygen is part of the water molecule ($H2O$) which makes life possible.

A plant is a living organism—a tree, shrub, herb, grass, fern, flower, vegetable, weed, or moss. Plants absorb water and inorganic or non-living substances through their roots. The green plant pigment captures the light. Plants manufacture their own food molecules using energy obtained from light.

Plants create nutrients in their leaves by photosynthesis, which is a process by which green plants and other organisms turn carbon dioxide and water into carbohydrates and oxygen. According to Wikipedia, carbon dioxide is a colorless, odorless gas vital to life on earth. It is a chemical compound made up of a carbon atom and two oxygen atoms.

Essential oils are found in the plant's flowers, leaves, resin, wood, roots, fruit, and seeds. The lavender angustifolia essential oil or true lavender is a colorless or pale-yellow liquid. It is sweet floral, herbaceous, and refreshing, with a slightly woody smell.

Understanding the typical chemical composition of an essential oil helps to provide a scientific understanding of its beneficial use. Here are true lavender's key chemical components.

Monoterpenes: analgesic, antiseptic, antiviral, decongestant, a tonic, stimulant, and hormone-like. Monoterpene alcohols: antibacterial, antifungal, antiviral, tonic, a stimulant, and sedative. They are the most beneficial and safest of all essential oil constituents. Monoterpene ketones: wound-healing, yet can act as a neurotoxin, which means they may impair nerve tissue function. They are analgesic and antiviral. Esters: antispasmodic, anti-inflammatory, calming and a tonic to the nervous system, antifungal, and sedative. Esters are generally safe to use and have low toxicity.

Essential oils have tiny molecular structures making them extremely potent and concentrated. Inhaling even a small amount of essential oil vapor can produce profound effects on the body, brain, and emotions. Knowing when to use more or less of an essential oil makes a huge difference and is the art of genuine aromatherapy.

Scientists are uncovering biological connections between humans and plants. Some research revealed that plant and human biology is much closer than once thought. A study of these similarities could help to reveal the biological basis of diseases.

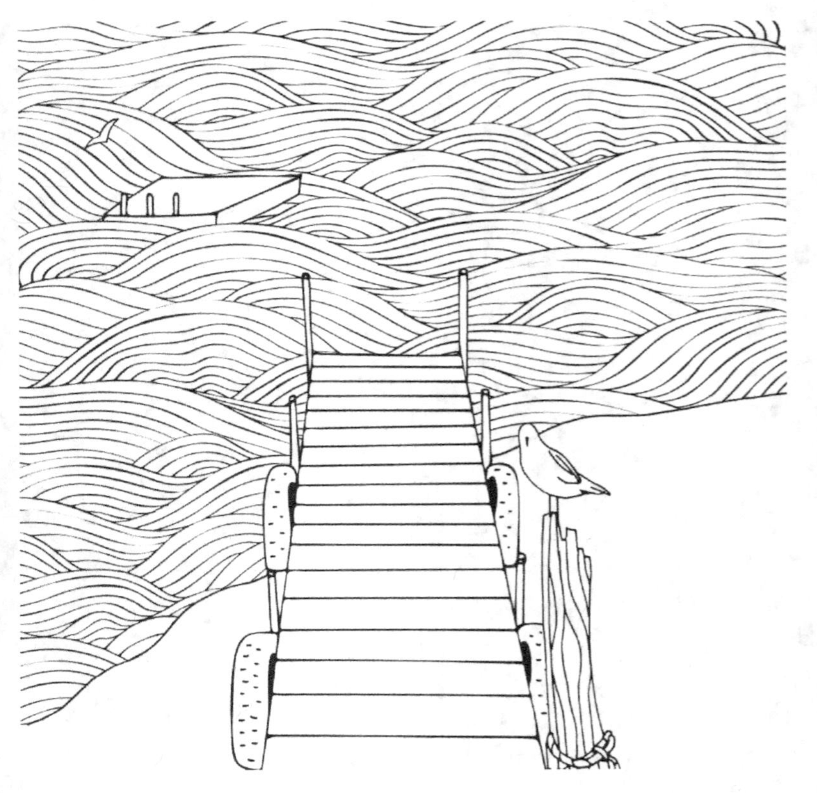

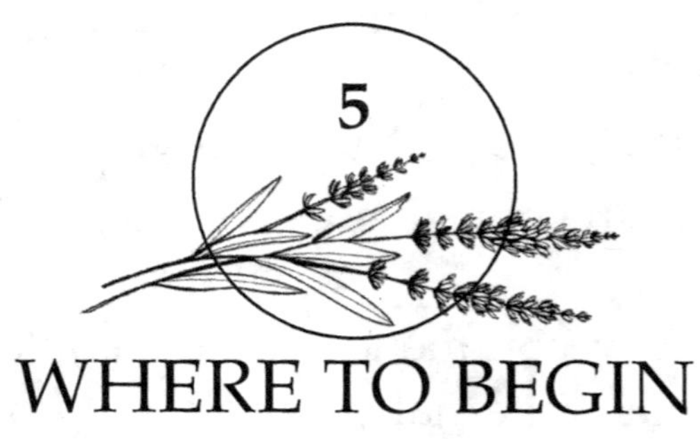

WHERE TO BEGIN

"But you, you foolish girl, you have gone home to a leaky castle across the sea to lie awake in linen smelling of lavender, and hear the nightingale, and long for me."

Edna St. Vincent Millay

Information on how to use essential oils found on the internet, social media, and in books can be confusing. Gaining the safest best data is a challenge. Take time to research and determine credibility.

One good source for sorting through practice advice is the National Association for Holistic Aromatherapy (NAHA). The organization educates health care practitioners and the general public on safe and responsible use of essential oils.

NAHA recommends that people not use oils internally "unless properly trained in the safety issues of doing so." Representatives of big essential oil companies may advocate internal use and often advertise their essential oil products as better than their competition because they're "therapeutic grade" or "certified pure therapeutic grade." These terms, used for marketing purposes, may not be backed by authority. Look for specific facts about the essential oil, its general use and safety.

It takes a while to obtain and understand how to apply essential oils. If you use retail companies that provide essential oil blends, be sure to read labels carefully and try a few to evaluate how they meet your support needs. Essential oils from grocery stores, health food stores, or pharmacy chains may be worth exploring, but what about quality? One way to determine quality is by comparing prices. For example, don't be fooled by an inexpensive price for rose essential oil which easily cost $50 for a 5 ml bottle.

After completing my aromatherapy training, I researched essential oils through books, classes, and on the internet. That was over ten years ago. Now there are many more places to find essential oils online. I read through each website, comparing information and prices, before settling on a few. Then I purchased one or two small bottles or samples of commonly used essential oils from these companies and compared them to each other. Most often the cheaper essential oils did not hold up. They smelled "off" after a short time.

In my studies, I was exposed to sixty-five quality essential oil aromas. Being scientific but leaning toward intuition and my sixth sense, I was able to determine which essential oils were of high quality. The nose knows!

The process I used took some investment of money and time but was a good learning experience. It is difficult to purchase a quality essential oil, even after studying them, without smelling and using the essential oil. Don't underestimate the value of aromatherapy education on your journey to use essential oils.

Special care and clear knowledge should be employed with essential oils on or around animals. Horses and dogs do fine with most oils. Cats should not be treated with essential oils. Reports about using them on cats are conflicting. It is better to avoid doing so. Be sure your cat does not get too close to the diffuser.

Lavender essential oil is not toxic, irritating, or sensitizing. It can be applied directly to the skin without diluting it. The safest way to apply lavender essential oil undiluted is to use a very small amount and see how you react. Each person's response will be different.

With essential oils, "less is more." In other words, increasing the amount of essential oil does not mean it will work better; usually it is the opposite. Adding just a little more lavender than needed can cause the reverse effect of restlessness instead of calm.

It is important not to use the same essential oil repeatedly in the same area on your skin, because you can become sensitive or allergic from overexposure. The allergy may appear as a minor breathing problem, hives, or the inability to smell the oil. Take an occasional break from your favorite essential oils.

Here is a list of "do nots" to consider: do not purchase undiluted essential oils without a dropper insert to restrict flow, do not use essential oils with a poorly identified label, do not use undiluted on the skin (lavender is an exception), placing a drop or two of undiluted essential oils in the palm of one hand and rubbing your hands together to inhale them is allowed, do not take essential oils internally unless directed by a trained professional with credible references, and finally, do not apply citrus essential oils before going out in the sun because they may cause the skin's sensitivity to sunlight to increase and the skin to become damaged. There are some exceptions with citrus essential oils and sun sensitivity. It depends on how the essential oil was obtained and the percentage of dilution.

Keep out of the reach of children. Use extra care with essential oils for sensitive individuals, children, pregnant women, and those with epilepsy, high blood pressure, or asthma. Store undiluted essential oils in dark-colored glass bottles in a cool place out of the sun. Transfer small amounts of essential oil remaining in a big bottle to a smaller bottle. This will avoid oxidation or deterioration, especially of citrus essential oils, because they oxidize quickly.

NAHA recommends per their website: If essential oil droplets accidentally get into the eye (or eyes), a cotton cloth or similar should be saturated with a fatty oil, such as olive or sesame, and CAREFULLY SWIPED OVER THE CLOSED LID, and/or immediately flush the eyes with cool water. Also if an essential oil causes dermal or skin irritation, apply a small amount of vegetable oil or cream to the area and discontinue use of essential oil or the product that caused the irritation. If a child appears to have swallowed several spoonfuls of essential oil, contact the nearest poison control unit. Keep the bottle for identification and encourage the child to drink whole or 2% milk. DO NOT try to induce vomiting.

When using an essential oil and water mixed without an emulsifier, the oils will not disperse evenly. Mix an emulsifier with your essential oils BEFORE you add them to your water base and blend well. A blend of one part emulsifier to one part essential oils is adequate. A highly diluted solution is safe to use without an emulsifier if you shake well each time.

Most essential oils, including lavender, are obtained by distillation. NAHA gives us a detailed explanation of how this is done. "…the plant material is placed upon a grid inside the still. Once inside, the still is sealed, and… steam or water/steam slowly breaks through the plant material to remove its volatile constituents. These volatile constituents rise upward through a connecting pipe that leads them into a condenser. The condenser cools the rising vapor back into liquid form. The liquid is then collected in a vehicle below the condenser. Since water and essential oil do not mix, the essential oil will be found on the surface of the water where it is siphoned off."

The aromatic water that remains after this distilling process is called a hydrosol. These hydrosols have wonderful healing properties and are like the essential oils but are far less concentrated. Lavender hydrosol is especially gentle, which makes it great for children.

Some essential oils may interfere with homeopathic remedies; check with your practitioner. Examples might be peppermint, eucalyptus, or tea tree.

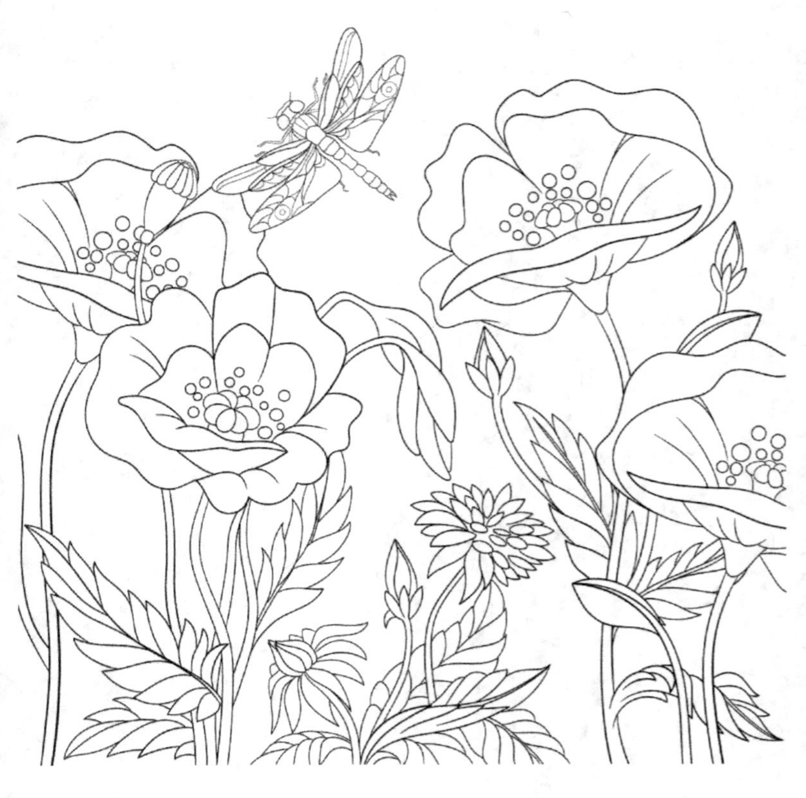

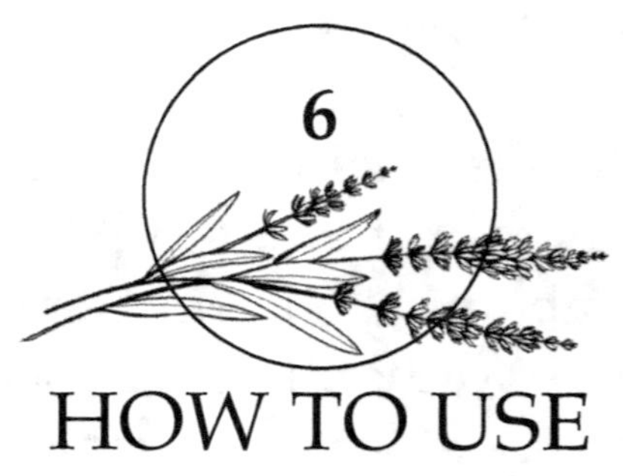

HOW TO USE

"When the light turns green, you go. When the light turns red, you stop. But what do you do when the light turns blue with orange and lavender spots?"

Shel Silverstein

The safest, most effective use of essential oils is to apply them diluted to the skin using carrier oil or water. They can also be diffused into the air. If taken orally or rectally, which is less common, they may not be as effective and should be used with consultation from a trained professional.

When you inhale an essential oil aroma, it is sensed by the olfactory nerve in the back of your nose and transported to the brain. The essential oil is absorbed into the bloodstream through the nasal mucous membrane. Your emotions are activated due to the direct impact on the primitive areas, or the limbic system. The influence of aroma on your psyche, along with its elusive ability to prevent illness, is not easy to measure, yet profound healing can be observed.

Essential oils and the vegetable-based carrier oils that are used to dilute and transport them are composed of fat-soluble dissolving molecules. These molecules or particles are easily absorbed into the skin. The essential oils enter the blood capillaries or passageways. Some examples of carrier oils used in aromatherapy are coconut, olive, grapeseed, sweet almond oil, and jojoba oil.

Many people buy essential oils and find that using them is not simple. Here are basic ways to fit essential oils into your busy life.

Hold an open bottle of essential oil (that has a dropper insert) and gently move the bottle closer to your nose. Breathe in slowly, then take a deep breath.

Place a drop of undiluted essential oil in the palm of one hand, then rub your hands together. Cup your palms about your mouth and nose and breathe in.

Put a drop or two of undiluted essential oil on/in an aromatherapy pendant, bracelet, or earrings to enjoy the aroma throughout the day.

Use a few drops of undiluted essential oil on a tissue, cotton ball, or potpourri. Put it at your bedside while sleeping, throughout your home, carry it with you in your purse or wallet, or place in your car's air vent. Avoid using lavender or other relaxing oils while driving. Use peppermint, lemongrass or rosemary to keep alert. Use rose, vanilla, orange, cinnamon, fir or spruce in your home in a potpourri of dried flowers to create a welcome ambience.

Place several drops of undiluted essential oils in a diffuser. An ultrasonic diffuser uses air, water, and ultrasonic vibrations to disperse the oil into the air. A fine mist is sent out, creating a humidifying effect. The oil molecules remain bound in the air for hours while the oil's therapeutic value or its ability to help is kept intact. You can use two or three essential oils that go well together or a single essential oil. (Most essential oils in this book are good for diffusing. A few drops are all you need.)

Apply essential oils diluted in a carrier oil to skin areas, and rub in lightly. A dilution of about 2% is recommended for a full-body massage. A dilution of 5-10% is effective for application to smaller skin areas for specific problems.

Apply diluted essential oils to the soles of your feet. The bottoms of your feet contain some of the largest pores in the body, causing the oils to be absorbed in a few minutes and travel your body's energy channels.

Dilute one to several drops of essential oil in a few tablespoons of carrier oil and pour into a warm bath or a foot soak. Lightly stir the water before stepping in. The oils absorb through your skin and by inhalation. (Take care not to slip.)

Place a diluted blend of three to five of your favorite oils on pulse points and wear like a perfume. You can also use a single essential oil like rose, jasmine, patchouli, or ylang ylang because their beautiful lasting aromas stand on their own as a perfume. It's nice to wear a natural perfume instead of applying man-made perfumes that may contain harmful chemicals. A dilution of 10-50% can be used on pulse points (behind ears, wrist, elbow fold, chest).

Mix essential oils with distilled or tap water in a glass spray bottle, then shake before spraying as an air freshener (use a fine mister). Spray into the air and away from your face.

Stir into a bucket of water several drops of essential oils like lavender, lemon, orange, or pine to clean. For a sweeter floral aroma, add a few drops of ylang ylang. Or use these oils in a large plastic spray bottle and shake well before spraying.

Work in a ventilated space. Pour oils at eye level above a table or desk protected by a mat. Keep a moist cloth handy to wipe your hands and the bottles. Do not touch your face, especially your eyes, when handling essential oil containers.

Tip the essential oil bottle slowly, watching and counting each drop as it goes into the bottle. The thinner oils will flow fast (tip the bottle gently) and the thicker oils will flow slowly. Do not worry if you get one or two drops more or less of an essential oil. But do concentrate on being accurate. Take your time. Make a reference card for your creations to include all the ingredients, number of drops for each essential oil, date mixed, and if desired, give it a name.

When you create a blend of essential oils, your hands and electromagnetic energy field are yours alone and influence your results. Even if another person uses the exact same ingredients and technique, the perfume will be different for each person. You have probably noticed how the perfume you wear smells different on someone else. It is because a person's individual body chemistry interacts with it and produces a different aroma.

Remember, the most important ingredient in any essential oil formula is love. Always handle oils when you are in a quiet, peaceful mood. Avoid mixing essential oils if you are tired, anxious, or rushed. The blend you make will reflect your feelings. Allow a positive spirit to infuse your creation. Your body, mind, and soul will thank you.

A guide for diluting essential oils:

ESSENTIAL OIL (number of drops per carrier oil)	CARRIER OIL (amount of carrier oil in milliliters (ml) or in drops to dilute essential oils)
1/2-1	1 ml (20 drops)
1-5	5 ml (100 drops)
2-10	10 ml (200 drops)
3-15	15 ml (300 drops)
4-20	20 ml (400 drops)
5-25	25 ml (500 drops)
6-30	30 ml (600 drops)

The PERCENT of dilution for all of the above uses the most drops per carrier oil at 5% (based on 20 drops = 1 ml). For a lesser % use the lesser number of drops per milliliter.	To find the % always divide the drops used by the drops per ml. For example, if you use 7 drops per 10 ml (or 200 drops) it is 7/200 or 0.035 which is 3.5 %.

I received my diploma in Aromatherapy and Oriental Medicine from The Institute of Traditional Herbal Medicine and Aromatherapy. The course included instruction on essential oil production, quality, science, safety, application methods, absorption routes, an in-depth study of sixty-five essential oils, aromatic acupressure level 1, and aromatherapy in clinical practice. The courses were conducted at the Heal Center in Atlanta, GA.

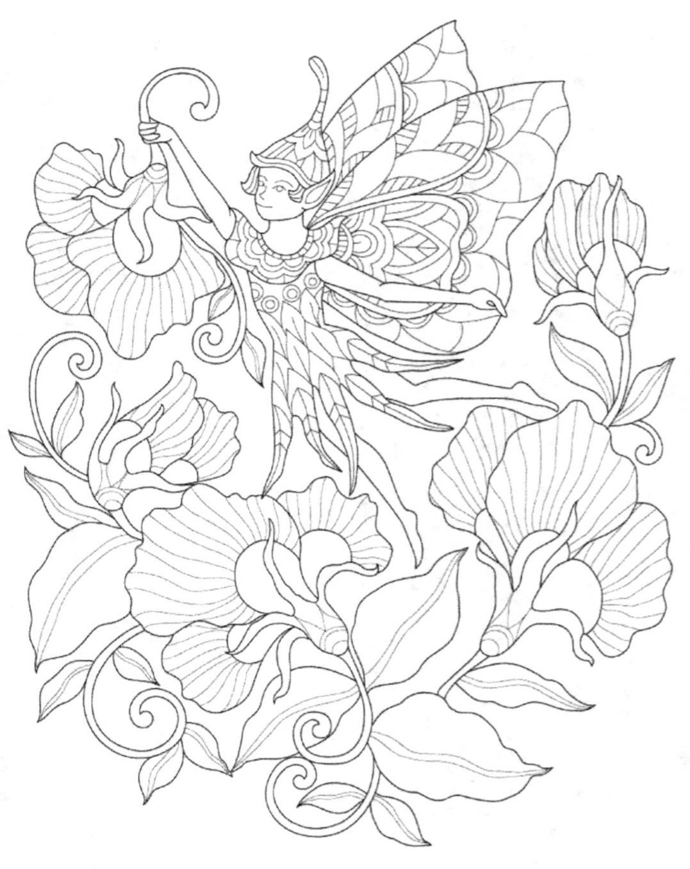

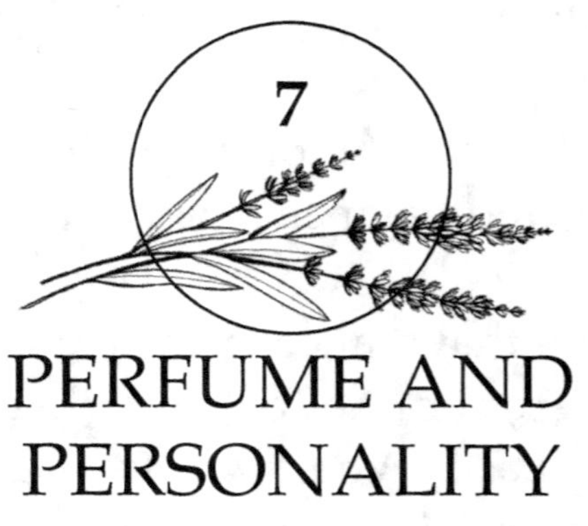

PERFUME AND PERSONALITY

"I think a fragrance is more of a signature than even what you wear — something you'll remember more down the road than a shirt."

Ryan Reynolds

To create a perfume using lavender as its center for balance is about combining science, art, and intuition. Make it as individual as you are, to fit your personality and fragrance preference. For example, you may enjoy the sensual florals of jasmine, ylang ylang, and rose mixed with the woodsy forest aromas of cedarwood, oakmoss, and fir. I do. Lavender enters these oils with its top to middle note to enhance and balance a blend as desired.

The notes that make up a perfume are divided between the top, middle or heart, and the base. When you create an aromatic essential oil mixture, the notes will evaporate at different stages. At the start of the fragrance you may smell all three notes. They will cycle through over time, revealing less of the top, then less middle, and finally you will smell the base or what is referred to as the dry down aroma. This way the blend remains pleasant, lasts longer, and smells different as the oils fade away from your skin.

You can modify a blend. It depends on the type of essential oil or absolute (obtained by solvent extraction) and the number of drops used. A perfume scent can be crafted with essential oils similar to your own liking. Combine top, middle, and base notes that would be happy together and willing to share their spirit with you. It's fun to enhance the splendor and magic of your personal scent by pouring it into a beautiful crystal perfume bottle.

The notes of a fragrance often sit at a standard percent when creating a complex blend of three or more essential oils. Top notes may be up to 25 percent, middle notes around 50 percent or more, and base notes similar to the top ranging from 10 to 25 percent depending on their tenacity. Often less is better for a strong base note that may take over the other aromas.

It's best to gradually add the essential oil drops into a glass container. Gently swirl them clockwise. Make a note of the number of drops as you add them. Allow some time for them to meld smelling as you go. It may take a few days before you know how much to add for each essential oil before your desired aroma emerges. Do not dilute the essential oils until they have had time to get to know each other first. Use recommended dilution ratios for safety.

The five elements used in clinical practice in traditional Chinese medicine are wood, fire, earth, metal (air), and water. The elements relate to the different qualities and functions of the body. Wood is liver and gallbladder. Fire is heart, pericardium, small intestine, sympathetic and parasympathetic, and the nervous system. Earth is stomach, spleen, and digestive processes. Metal (air) is lungs, colon, and skin. Water is kidney, bladder, bones, and the endocrine system.

The elements are also related to emotions. Wood is flexibility and growth. Fire is relationships and love. Earth is empathy and care. Metal (air) is self-worth and the ability to let go. Water is willpower and courage.

Each essential oil will bring elements of its own "life force" qualities to the blend.

When they join together, a true essence or perfume will be infused with bene-fits beyond what one single essential oil could provide.

The perfume combination below is a sim-ple example of how essential oils may be mixed in a signature scent. It consists of five essential oils: petigrain, lavender, ylang ylang, cedarwood, and oakmoss. The aromatic ingredients you choose for your own blend will depend on your in-dividual desires.

A TOP NOTE tends to be fresh and sharp when it first hits the nose. It lasts about thirty minutes on your body and lifts the spirit. Orange and lemon are often used as top citrus notes. To avoid any sun-sen-sitive skin reaction, petigrain essential oil is a good option. It is distilled from the leaves of the bitter orange plant and is not phototoxic. Petigrain also provides some intensity and staying power for a top note.

PETIGRAIN (Citrus aurantium supsp. Armara.) is an evergreen tree with long spines and fragrant flowers. Its oil is steam-distilled from the leaves of the bitter orange. The oil is a pale-yellow-amber color and has a pleasant fresh-floral and herbaceous aroma. It is reported to help with digestive, nervous, respiratory, and skin care. It is non-toxic and non-sensitizing. Use it for emotional nourishment and to improve your intellect. Allow its connection to the fire element to unite your heart and mind to better visualize your path and provide personal protection as you journey.

A MIDDLE NOTE is literally at the heart or center, not unlike our own physical heart. It helps balance the top and base notes and may last up to three hours on your body. Choose lavender to act as a top to middle note, and ylang ylang as a middle to base note for a floral-herbal aroma. Lavender does not have the high intensity of ylang ylang, but they join in creating a pleasant, lasting bouquet.

LAVENDER (Lavandula angustifolia) is an aromatic evergreen sub-shrub with lance-shaped leaves. The oil is steam-distilled from the freshly cut flowering tops and stalks. It has a colorless to pale yellow hue with a sweet floral herbaceous aroma and a balsamic-woody undertone. LAVENDER ABSOULTE (Lavandula angustifolia) from France is a dark-brown, viscous liquid with a rich deep floral, herbaceous, honeyed, and woody aroma. The oil is obtained by solvent extraction. It is my favorite lavender and works well in a perfume. Lavender is reported to help with skin, muscles and joints, nervous, reproductive, and respiratory care. The oil is safe and non-toxic. Use it to ease your soul, mind, and body. Let its bond with the metal (air) element remind you of your true divine self.

YLANG YLANG (Cananga odorata var. genuina) is a tall tropical evergreen tree. Its oil is produced from steam and water distillation of the freshly picked flowers. The oil is pale yellow and has a powerful floral sweet aroma. It is reported to help with circulatory, nervous, reproductive, and skin care. This oil is safe and non-toxic. Excessive use may cause head-aches and nausea. Apply it to chase away angry feelings and replace them with a sweet, sensual sense of peace. Let its affection for the water element resonate with the water in your body to arouse your sensual, loving nature.

A BASE NOTE gives the blend depth, warmth, and staying power so after three to four hours its aroma will still linger on your body. Choose cedarwood atlas and oakmoss for base notes to create a woodsy forest scent. Cedarwood does not have the high intensity of oakmoss, but they bind to each other and create a strong fragrant floor.

CEDARWOOD (Cedrus atlantica) is a tall majestic evergreen tree. Its oil is produced from steam-distilled wood stumps, sawdust, or wood chips. The oil is a thick, deep-amber color and has a sweet, tenacious-woody aroma. It is reported to help with lymphatic, nervous, respiratory, urinary, and skin care. It is non-toxic and non-irritating. Use it to dispel fear, provide strength, and deepen your spiritual nature. Allow its affinity for the fire element to increase your confidence to become a tower of strength for those around you in need.

OAKMOSS (Evernia prusnatri) is a complex fungi-algae lichen, not a moss, that grows on the branches of oak trees. Its oil is solvent-extracted and vacuum-distilled. The oil is a greenish-black color and has a seashore and yet sweet earthy pervasive scent. It is reported to help with nervous, respiratory, digestive, and skin care. ***It may cause skin irritation and should be avoided when pregnant or have neurological disorders. It is best mixed in small amounts and well diluted. Use it to enter the forest or escape to the sea and to increase your personal prosperity. Relate to its earth element in the digestion of your hungers and in your concern for the welfare of others.

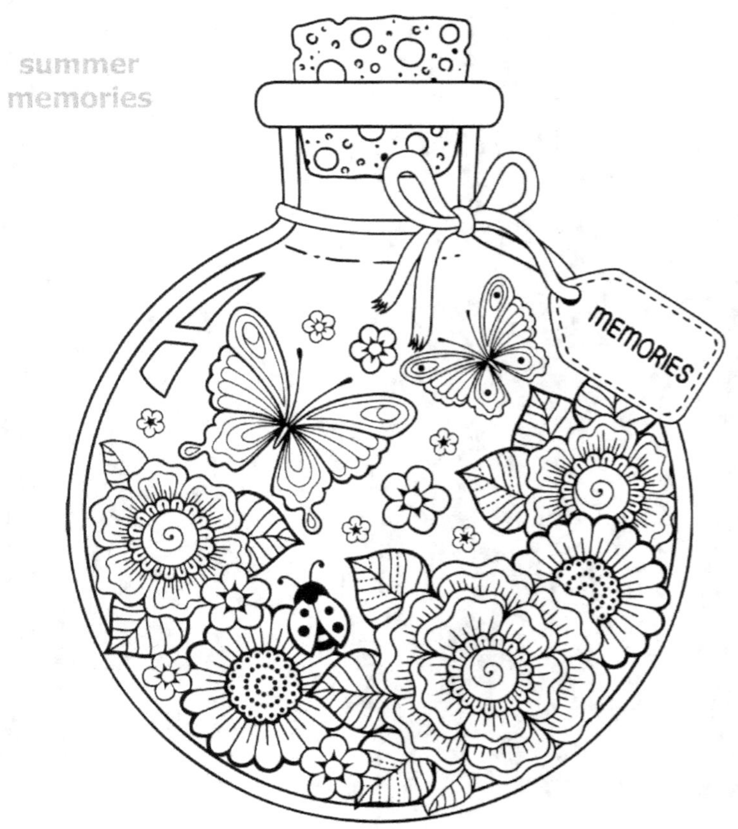

summer
memories
MEMORIES

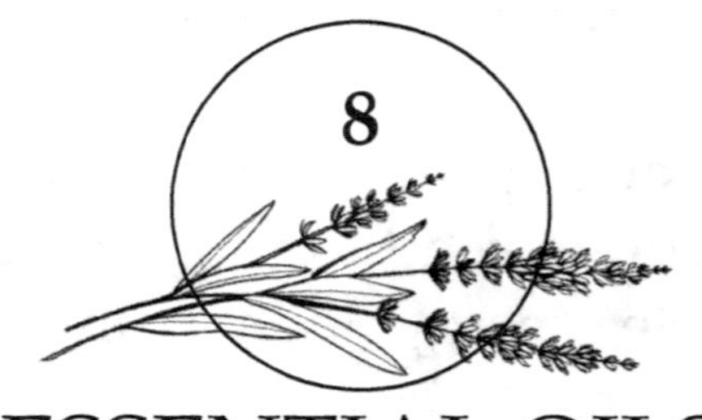

ESSENTIAL OILS
ENERGY AND HEALTH

"Why natural oils? Why not anything that smells nice, weather it is natural or synthetic? The answer is simply that synthetic or inorganic substances do not contain any 'life force': they are not dynamic. Everything is made of chemicals, but organic substances like essential oils have a structure which only Mother Nature can put together. They have a life force, an additional impulse which can only be found in living things."

Robert Tisserand,
The Art of Aromatherapy

The following are twenty-four essential oils described in terms of their perfume note, energy, aroma, and healthy support.

ESSENTIAL OIL	NOTE	ENERGY	AROMA	HEALTHY SUPPORT
Black Pepper	Middle	Move Stimulate	Fresh dry-woody warm-spicy	anemia, digestion, tired aching muscles, joints, feeling cold
Cedarwood (atlas)	Base	Succeed Strengthen	Sweet-woody	lymph flow, anxiety, coughs, oily skin
Chamomile (roman)	Middle	Voice Gentle	Tea leaf-like	digestion, migraines, headaches, insomnia, PMS (premenstrual symptoms), dry skin
Cinnamon	Middle	Perk-up Renew	Warm-spicy	bacterial and viral infection, stomach spasms, diarrhea, nausea and vomiting, nervous depression
Clary sage	Middle-Base	Clarify Uplift	Floral herbaceous	depression, mental activity, tension, menstrual cycle, childbirth, menopause, asthma, spasms, sweating, oily skin

Cypress	Middle	Learn Harmonize	Refreshing	varicose veins, feeling overburdened, PMS, coughs, sweating, oily skin
Frankincense	Base	Meditate Relax	Fresh terpene-like	anxiety, restlessness, shallow breathing, insomnia, dry skin, scars, wrinkles
Geranium	Middle	Stabilize Healthful	Green leafy-rosy	cellulite, edema, eczema, burns, wounds, depression, headaches, anxiety, PMS, menopause, combination skin, workaholics
Ginger	Middle	Encourage Active	Warm woody-spicy	high cholesterol, inflammation, nausea, fever, morning and motion sickness, cold hands and feet, poor circulation, arthritis, coughs, lower back pain, tired muscles
Jasmine	Base	Desire Sensual	Rich warm floral	nervous anxiety, restlessness, depression, sexual relationships, emotional difficulty, apathy, PMS, fearfulness, dry skin

Lavender	Middle	Comfort Balance	Floral herbaceous	burns, acne, boils, sunburn, inflammation, muscle aches and pains, stress of any kind, anxiety, agitation, fear, insomnia, depression, migraines, headaches, PMS, colds, flu, difficult breathing, itching and scratching, insect bites, palpitations, high blood pressure
Lemon	Top	Sparkle Clean	Light sweet	plaque deposits, high cholesterol, varicose veins, low immunity, cold, flu, cellulite, mental fatigue, indecisiveness, aging skin, acne, warts, overheated ***do not use on skin before going in the sun

Marjoram (sweet)	Middle	Nurture Friendly	Warm-spicy camphor	bruises, high blood pressure, indigestion, constipation, gas, spasms, sprains, muscle and rheumatic pain, headaches, migraines, grief (only use a short time), cold, flu, coughs, PMS
Niaouli	Middle	Medicinal Therapeutic	Sweet-camphor	headaches, cough, cold, minor burns, bruises, muscle aches and pains, arthritis, acne, boils
Oakmoss	Base	Ocean Material	Sweet-forest & seashore	inflammation, infections, low immunity, wounds, mucous congestion *** may cause sensitivity in some individuals
Orange (sweet)	Top	Cheerful Open-hearted	Fresh citrus	upset stomach, spasms, constipation, gas, swollen tissues, anxiety, insomnia, mild depression, nervousness, aging or calloused skin *** may be phototoxic

Patchouli	Base	Hypnotic Grounded	Spicy-woody balsamic	sores, scars, fungal and parasitic skin infections, depression, anxiety, excessive mental activity, fatigue, abdominal distention, overthinking, worry
Peppermint	Middle	Inspire Quick-thinking	Grassy-minty	spasms, tension headaches, migraines, bruises, muscle joint pain, fungal and bacterial infection, nerve pain, stomach upset, diarrhea, gas, nausea, vomiting, travel sickness, congested lymph, poor concentration, fatigue, nervousness, colds, inferiority *** do not use on the face, especially the nose of infants and small children
Petitgrain	Top	Revitalize Intellectual	Fresh-floral woody-herbaceous	indigestion, exhaustion, stress, depression, insomnia, irritability, skin blemishes

Pine	Middle	Awaken Positive	Pine fresh sweet	muscle aches and pains, fatigue, nervous exhaustion, psychological stress, weakness, colds, cough, sinus congestion
Rose	Middle-Base	Love Emotional	Sweet warm rich floral	soul, mind, body, and spirt, depression, palpations, irritability, anger, despair, frustration, insomnia, fear, sorrow, PMS, mature dry sensitive skin, inflammation, emotional wounds, grief, sexual relationships
Rosemary	Middle	Youthful Invigorate	Clean-woody-balsamic	cardiac fatigue, palpations, low blood pressure, extremity circulation, gallbladder and liver problems, stiff overworked muscles, nervous debility, poor concentration, headaches, coughs, sinus congestion, hair growth, dandruff

| Vetiver | Base | Centering Earthy | Heavy-woody-root-like | arthritis, muscle pain, stress, insomnia, depression, anxiety, physical, mental, and emotional burnout, hormone imbalance, menopause, PMS, skin connective tissue, stretch marks after childbirth, poor appetite, weight loss, nutrient malabsorption |
| Ylang ylang | Middle-Base | Passionate Peaceful | Soft balsamic floral | epileptic seizures, palpations, high blood pressure, rapid heartbeat and breathing, shock, anxiety, anger, nervous depression, stress, frustration, sexual inadequacy, mood swings, PMS, hair split ends, dry or oily skin *** do not use in excess may cause nausea and headache |

REFERENCES

Heal Center
https://healcenteratlanta.com/

National Association for Holistic Aromatherapy
https://naha.org/

New Directions Aromatics
http://www.newdirectionsaromatics.com

Abundant health
http://www.abundanthealth4u.com

The National Center for Biotechnology Information
https://www.ncbi.nlm.nih.gov/pmc/articles/PMC5206475/citedby/

<u>The Complete Guide to Aromatherapy,</u> Salvatore Battaglia

<u>Aromatherapy for the Soul</u>, Valerie Ann Worwood

<u>Aromatherapy for Healing the Spirit</u>, Gabriel Mojay

<u>Magical Aromatherapy</u>, Scott Cunningham

<u>The Art of Aromatherapy</u>, Robert B. Tisserand

<u>Essence & Alchemy</u>, Mandy Aftel

<u>Perfume: The Art & Craft of Fragrance</u>, Karen Gilbert

About Susan Brougher

Susan gained technical and creative writing skills through her life work and experiences. Her varied background as a Registered Nurse spanned Hospital, Army Nurse Corps, Developmental & Behavioral, Environmental, Nursing & Personal Care Homes, and Home Health. She is a Registered Aromatherapist and a Healing Touch Practitioner-A. Susan writes, "Words form in our thoughts and travel in our blood the issue of life. They begin long before they fill blank pages and they live long after the book is closed." Look for her on Amazon, Goodreads, LinkedIn, and Pinterest. She welcomes your comments at susanspen1@gmail.com